Jyotirmoy Deb

Everyday Healthy

Contents

1

Author

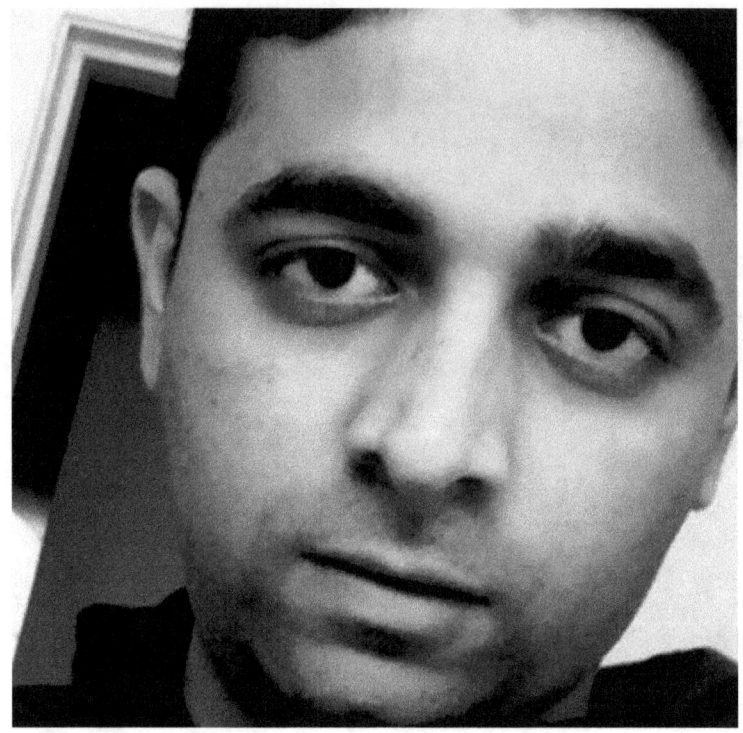

I am Jyotirmoy. I am an IT Engineer by Profession with a masters and bachelors in Computer Science.I am a programmer and have worked in several reputed IT companies over 10 years.

In my spare time I write Ebooks and do content marketing as a hobby.I have my own online portal which is an online market place for digital contents e.g Photos,Tutorial Videos, Ebooks. Please check my URL *www.theprecisecontent.com.*

I realize that the good things about life should be shared with everyone and internet is the platform. To express my feelings and experiences with the help of digital contents e.g. photos , videos and Ebooks make a direct effect on the readers and viewers.

I love what I do and always enjoy to spend as much time as possible on it.Hope you will like this book and recommend others.

2

Introduction

Being Healthy has become an integral part of our life. In todays world we can't afford to make unhealthy choices. In this new age of information we have to withstand with excessive stress every single day.To maintain a work-life balance and a good health is a challenge for many people.

In this book I have highlighted twenty different very important habits which are guaranteed to secure healthy living in day-to-day basis.These habits I developed from my own failures, mistakes and experiences.The more important thing rather than trying to follow these habits is to get concerned about the fact that we are getting exposed to many different situations everyday, some require intense mental or physical involvement. Knowingly or unknowingly we accomplish work and exert energy.Some times they have fruitful outcomes , sometimes not.Its extremely important to perform some activities explicitly to regain that loss.

These important habits are guaranteed to keep us healthy ,active , fresh and full of energy.My purpose to write this book is to acquaint the reader with the gain or positive outcomes by performing these habits.

Our lives are occupied by many different activities. Some of them ask for serious dedication and commitments from us and we can't avoid them such as raising our kids , maintaining grades at school, performing at work place. The amount of free time we get for ourselves is decreasing . In future I am afraid someday we may have to forget our existence.

3

chapter 1 : "Prioritizing Good Sleep is Good Self Love"

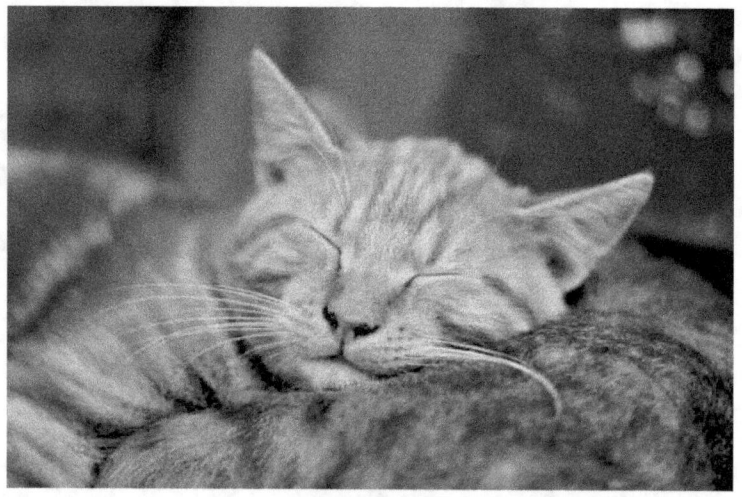

"sleep well"

Healthy habits may be applied based on Gender , Age Group or activity wise e.g Food Habit , Sleeping Habit etc. In this book I have generalized and highlighted all the habits which are common to all and can be followed easily.

The very first one is to develop a sleeping habit for at least 7-8 hours a day at least.We observe and experience different things through our eyes everyday.Some experiences are satisfactory , some are not.These experiences have an effect on our brain.If you don't give proper rest , you may encounter serious mental health problem e.g Anxiety , Stress Disorder. Some researchers have declared that less amount of sleep reduces life span.People who sleep less die early.

If you are not able to make a 7-8 hours of sleep at a stretch then develop a habit to fulfill in installments.To have a good and sound sleep is an important criteria for a healthy life.We can't skip that.

How to get better Sleep :

1. Early Rise and Early Bed : The best practice is to wake up early lets say 5am and going to bed at 9pm at night. Waking up early and exposing body to natural sunlight is a healthy habit.

You will get time to do some exercise and proper breakfast.It also helps to keep in sync with your body's natural sleep-wake cycle.

2. Exercise in Day : Join a health club and do vigorous exercise in the day time under exposure to natural sunlight. This helps to create an urge for sound sleep at night.

3. Surroundings : Create your own surroundings before

you sleep e.g maintaining low noise , cool room temperature , comfortable bed etc.At night it is recommended to sleep away from bright light for better sleep.

4. Avoid alcohol , nicotine or caffein : Avoid any alcohol ,nicotine or caffein before sleep. These elements disrupt sleep.You may get anxiety attack or panic attack in the middle of sleep and that won't be a pleasant experience I am sure.

5. Meal : Eating big or spicy meals can cause discomfort from indigestion that can make it hard to sleep. If you can, avoid eating large meals for two to three hours before bedtime.

Over Sleep :

Oversleep(sometimes also known as *hypersomnia*) is also not good for health. This is an abnormal behavior. It can happen from many different reasons. But if someone is suffering from this problem then it needs to be controlled.Some of the serious problems happen from oversleeping are ,

1. Higher Risk of having stroke
2. Infertility
3. Heart Disease
4. Cognitive impairment
5. Depression
6. Tendency to become over-weight or Obese

Nearly every human being on earth has some sort of sleeping

disorder.If you have some problem while sleeping ,my best advice is to contact to your doctor.Its important to have a routine check-up with your doctor immediately and save yourself from further problems.

4

Chapter 2: "Water is your Best Friend "

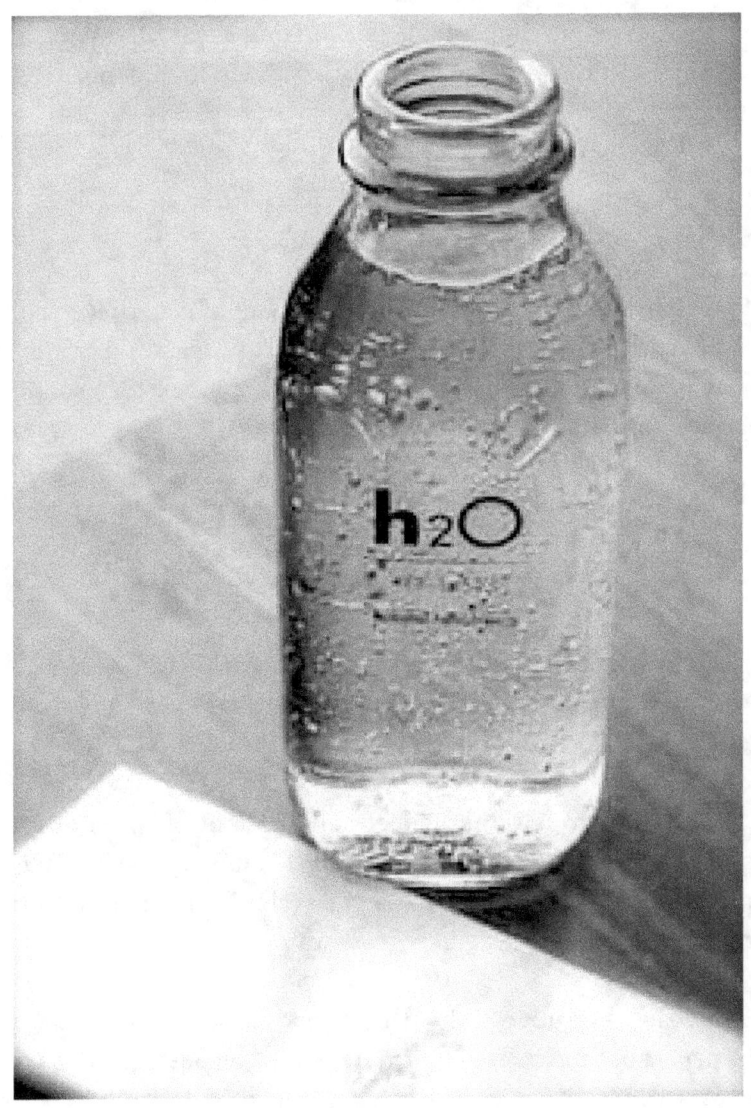

"Drink Drink Drink"

Water plays an important role in our life. Drinking a good amount of water surprisingly has the following positive outcomes.

Advantages :

1.Healthy Heart : Drinking a good amount of water save you to die from heart attack.A person drinking 5 glasses of water a day has 42% less chance to die from heart attack than some one who is drinking less than 2 glasses of water.

2.Motivate -Hydrate : Less amount of water in body can cause dehydration resulting into loss of energy.Dehydration leads to muscle fatigue, dizziness and other symptoms.

3.Healthy Skin : Drinking good amount of water over a week time period helps to maintain healthier skin.Your skin gets cleaned-up and starts glowing.

4.Metabolism : Drinking a certain amount of water after meal is an important habit for good digestion.Body needs water to digest food and water plays a vital role. People may suffer from constipation for drinking lass water.

5.Reduced Cancer Risk : Drink good amount of water over the period of time can reduce colon cancer , bladder cancer and breast cancer.

6.Exercise : Drinking water is a must while exercising. Muscle needs constant support of water. Scarcity of water may result into dehydration and muscle fatigue during exercise.

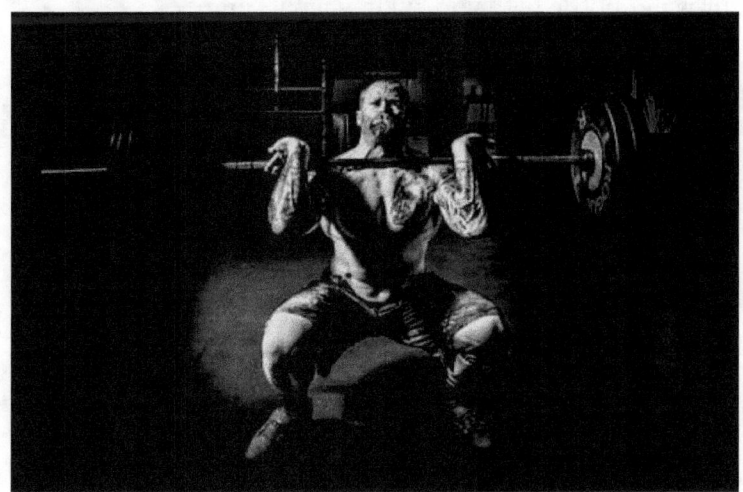

While Work-out you need Water

Water also removes toxic substances from the body and keep our body Kool and calm.There are several other benifits of drinking water.

How to regularize "Drinking Water" Habit :

So the question is how can we make drinking water a consistent habit. Here are some solutions.

1.Carry a water Bottle : Always carry a bottle wherever you go. When you are at work place ,or school or any where carry your water bottle with you.Fill it when its empty.

2.Set a timer : You can set a timer at your desktop , laptop , watch or cell phone at a certain interval for drinking water. If you have a habit of forgetting ,timer is a must.

3.Raplace with water : Normally we have a tendency to drink coffee , soda or alcohol. Its always better to replace them with water.

There is no replacement of water.Developing a habit of drinking water is a must.Water makes up about 60-70% of our body, and is present in our cells, tissues and organs. From lubricating the joints to protecting the spinal cord and other sensitive tissues, regulate body temperature, drinking water is absolutely essential for our body in order to function properly.

Chapter 3: "Eat Good Feel Good"

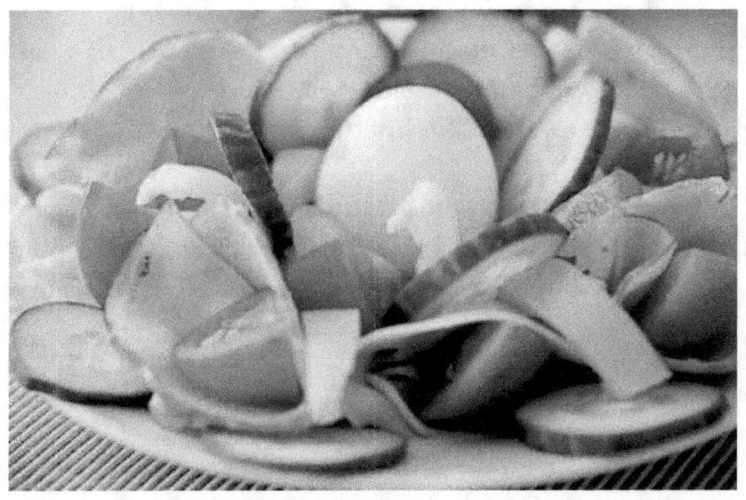

"A healthy man is a wealthy man". A good eating habits always promote a good health.Remember those moments in life when you had a good time. You enjoyed those moments only because you were healthy. We can not control everything in life but we can definitely control what we eat.Good food habits determine our future. Successes of life can't be enjoyed and shared if we don't have a good Mental and Physical health.

Here are some good food habits I would like to share.

1) Eat Vegetables and Fruits : The most important eating habit is to concentrate on fresh vegetables and fruits.These are definitely healthy diet.An approximate of 2.5 cups of vegetable and 2 cups of fruits give you around 2000 calories.Target Green, orange, red, blue/purple and yellow produce. The nutrients, fiber and other compounds in these foods may help protect against certain types of cancer and other diseases. Legumes, rich in fiber, count as vegetables, though are moderately high in calories, are also good for health.

2) Eating Healthy whole grains is a must : Whole grains have a lower *glycemic index* maintaining our energy level for longer. Try to buy whole grain pasta , brown rice , oats from super market.

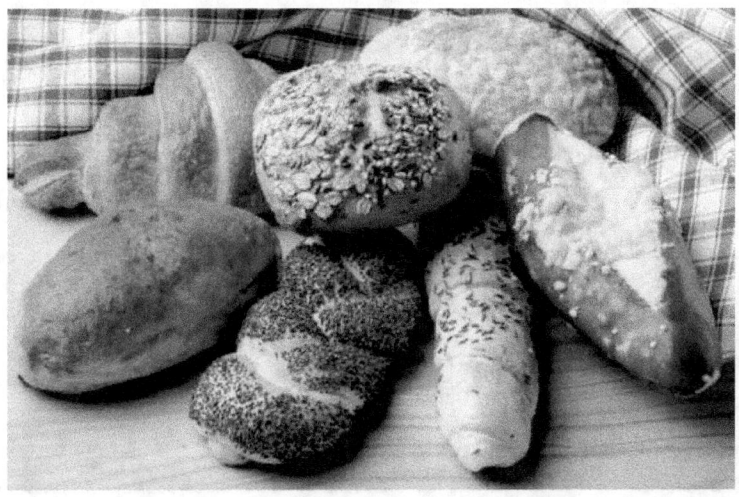

Made From whole grains

3) Switch to Healthy Unprocessed Food : Most of the packaged food we buy and eat are not healthy as they contain higher level of Fat , Salt and Sugar.We tend to buy them because it saves our cooking time and cheaper in price. Cooking Unprocessed food at home is a healthier option than packaged food.This means cooking with fresh vegetables, lean meat, eggs and milk and eating plenty of fruit, nuts and legumes.

4) Eat more Fish : Olive or canola oil , fatty fish , vegetables , avocados have unsaturated fat which help to reduce. heart disease risks largely because of the omega 3 polyunsaturated fat.

17

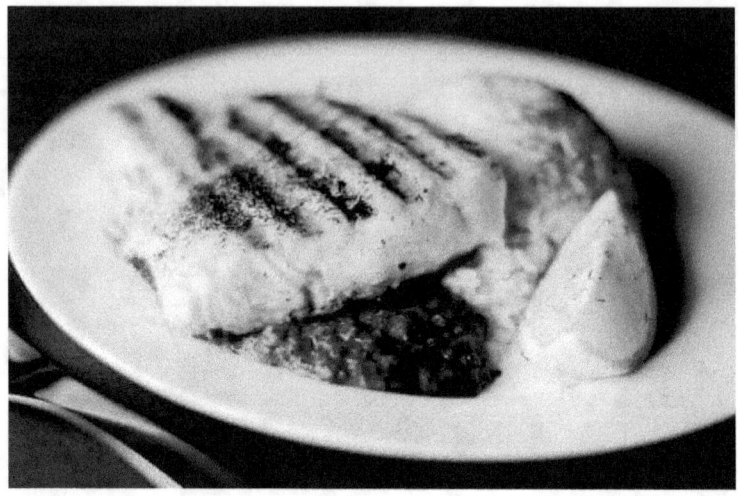

Fish

5) Reduce intake of red meat : Red meat contains saturated fat which has high cholesterol level and is bad for health.Switch to skinless poultry and low fat dairy products.

6) Alcohol-Nicotine-Caffeine : Intake of these three elements in large can lead to certain types of Cancer.Pregnant women should avoid intake of these elements. Intake of alcohol in moderate range is sometimes recommended by doctors as a part of social activity.Its recommended to avoid drinking soda e.g Coca Cola , Pepsi, energy drinks etc. these drinks contain caffeine which increase the chance of having heart disease , anxiety , depression and sleeping disorder.

Chapter 4 : "Wake up Early ,Work Out , Repeat"

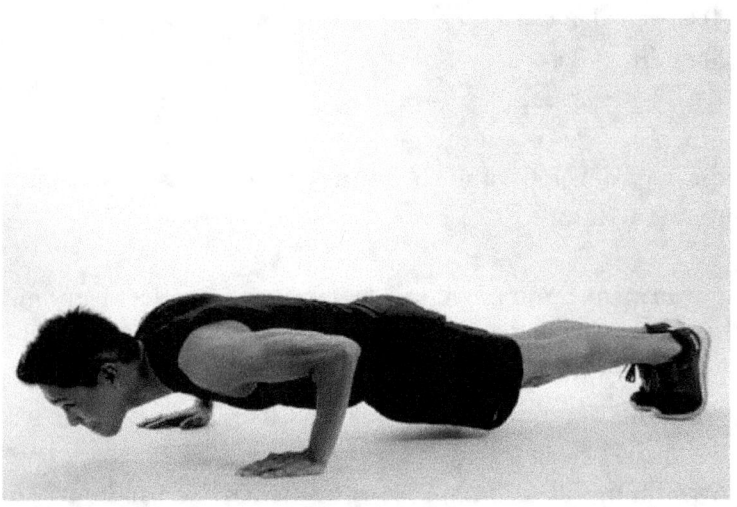

Physical Exercise is definitely one of the most important habit which we can't neglect to get a healthy life.Exercise maintains a lower risk of developing high blood pressure and diabetes.No matter your age or fitness level, these activities can help you get in shape and lower your risk for disease:

Strength Training : Strength training doesn't mean lifting heavy weights and pump your muscle.There are many people who are huge externally but lack core strength e.g. walking up hill or squats or chin ups will not be at-ease for them.This means they are weak internally.

Some of the important Core-Fitness Exercises are
1) Climbing Rope
2) Side Balance Crunch
3) Squat
4) Circle Plank
5) Sliding Pike

The most important thing is consistency and over the time these will develop your core fitness, your muscle strength, immune system.

Swimming : You might call swimming the perfect workout. The buoyancy of the water supports your body and takes the strain off painful joints so you can move them more fluidly. Swimming is good for individuals with arthritis because it's less weight-bearing.

Swimming can also improve your mental state and put you in a better mood. Water aerobics is another option. These help you burn calories and tone up.

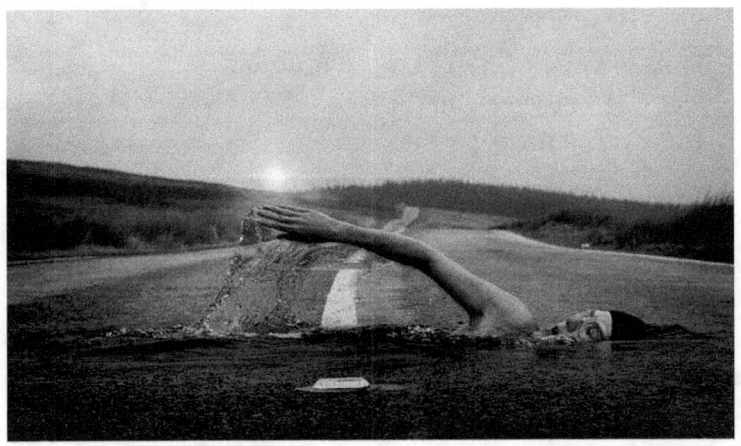

If you already don't know it,join some swimming club and get lessons.

Walking : Walking is simple, yet powerful. It can help you stay trim, improve cholesterol levels, strengthen bones, keep blood pressure in check, lift your mood, and lower your risk for a number of diseases (diabetes and heart disease, for example). A number of studies have shown that walking and other physical activities can even improve memory and resist age-related memory loss.

Free Hand Exercise : Freehand exercises have a tonic effect on the muscles and internal organs. They tone up the circulatory system and are beneficial in safeguarding the general health of the body. Advanced freehand exercises shape and muscularize the body.

Some of the more important are...

- **Push-Ups**
- **Dips Between Chairs Or On A Bench**
- **Rowing Between Chairs**
- **Handstand Push-Ups**
- **Sprinting, Racewalking, Lying Leg Curls**

Running : Running has a tremendous potential to maintain our heath.It has aesthetic benefits and mental health improvement.Running can not replace going to gym and workouts but we can keep it as a parallel activity.Following are the important positive outcomes from running.

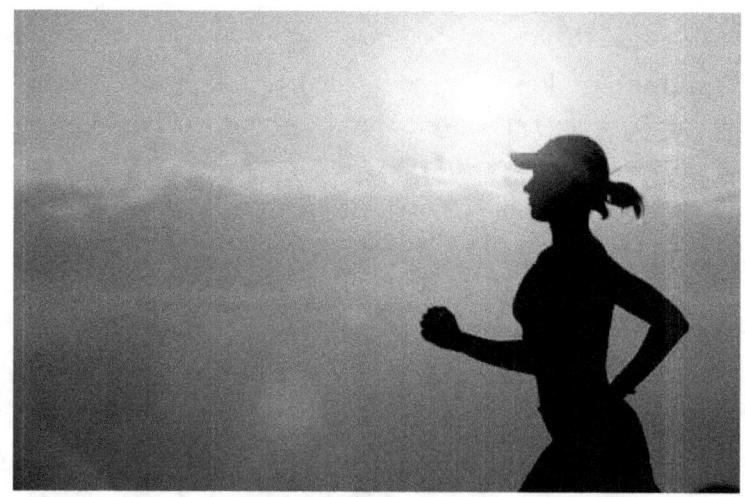

1) **Running Helps to Live Longer :** Researches has been done and it is proven that an individual running consistently lives longer than someone who is not.

2) **Running Keeps our energy level High :** hows that when we run, our brains pump out endocannabinoids, cannabis-like molecules that keep runners happy and hooked.

3) **Running helps to maintain belly-shape :** People who can run 35 or more miles a week are able to maintain flat belly in their middle age.

4) **Running help to gain Vitamin D**

5) **Running Burns Crazy Calories**

6) **Running Strengthen your bones**

7) **Running helps to fight with common colds**

Tai-chi : This Chinese martial art that combines movement and relaxation is good for both body and mind. In fact, it's been called "meditation in motion." is made up of a series of graceful movements, one transitioning smoothly into the next. Because the classes are offered at various levels, tai chi is accessible — and valuable — for people of all ages and fitness levels. "It's particularly good for older people because balance is an important component of fitness, and balance is something we lose as we get older.

Chapter 6 : Yoga and Meditation

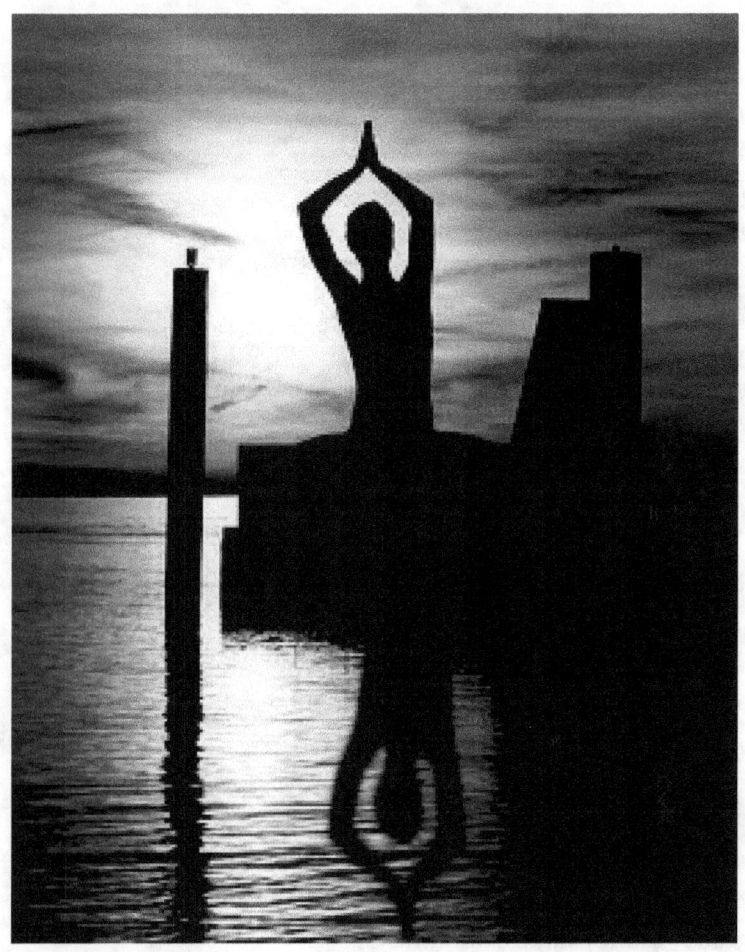

Yoga

Yoga is very old(probably 5000 years) Indian technique to breath
, stretch ,turns and other physical exercise. Yoga has immense
potential and has been accepted world wide. The science behind

yoga is not only to gain a level of fitness but it also to unfold the infinite potentials of the human mind and soul. The science of Yoga imbibes the complete essence of the Way of Life.

Benefits from Yoga

Here are some of the benefits from yoga. There are several other benifits.

1. Posture : Yoga is important to give our body a nice posture.The way we sit, sleep , walk everything can be effected from yoga.Wrong postures can create pain to neck ,shoulder , bone joints leading to arthritis.

2.Cardiovascuar : Yoga is also important to reduce the risk of heart-attack.It improves cardiovascular functionality. Studies have found that yoga practice lowers the resting heart rate, increases endurance, and can improve your maximum uptake of oxygen during exercise—all reflections of improved aerobic conditioning.

3.Blood Sugar : Yoga is very important to lower the level of blood sugar and reducing the amount of cholesterol there by reducing the chances of having diabetic problems such as heart attack , kidney failure ,blindness .

4.Nervous System : Yoga has tremendous power to control the body in unusual way.It has been found that "yogi"s of earlier days were able to control their body and nervous system using the power of yoga in a unusual manner.Consistent yoga definitely has an effect to control our nerves.

5. Better sleep : Another by-product of a regular yoga practice, studies suggest, is better sleep—which means you'll be less tired and stressed and less likely to have accidents.

6.Helps you focus: An important component of yoga is focusing on the present. Studies have found that regular yoga practice improves coordination, reaction time, memory, and even IQ scores. It improves problem solving ability , better concentration there by less likely to get distracted by external attraction.

Meditation

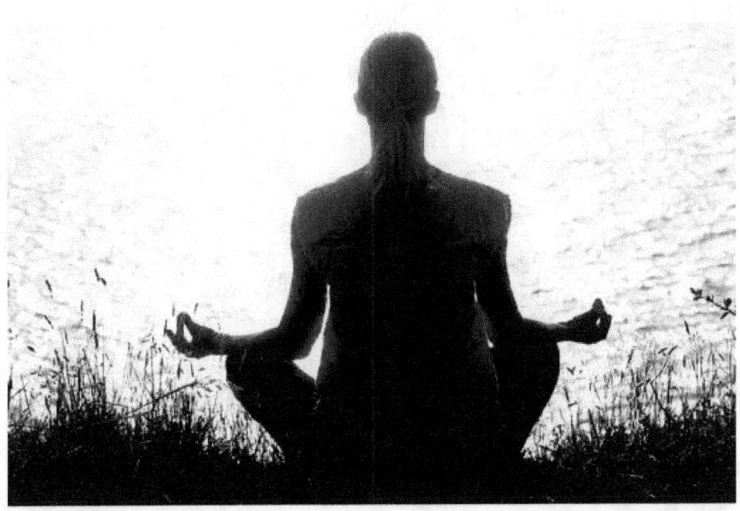

Meditation has become a part of life for many people , mostly those who suffer from mental instability because of some problem .Meditation helps to calm down ,relax your body and mind and connects your mind to a spiritual level.There are different ways of doing meditation by different people.Follow whichever is convenient for you.

Here are some Guaranteed Benefits from Meditation.
1. It reduces high blood pressure.
2. It removes body pains which happen from tension.
3. It improves our immune system.
4. It helps to increase body energy.
5. Improves Mental stability.
6. Improves Decision making ability.
7. Releases Anxiety.
8. Gives us happiness in our work.
9. Reduces Depression.
10. Helps to Reduce Panic Disorder.

1.

Chapter 5: Sports and Outdoors

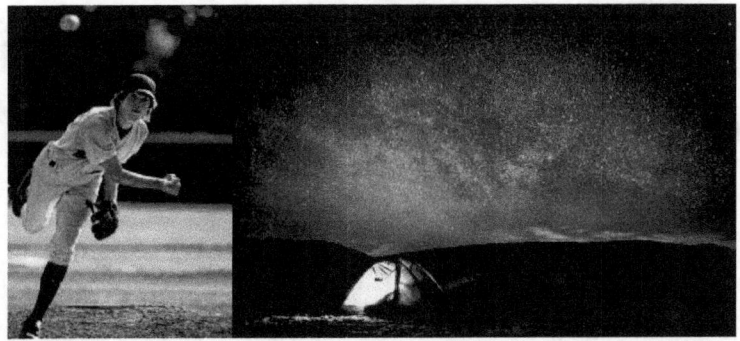

Fitness Exercises are definitely important. These give us energy , spirit and boost for gaining core strength. Sports and Outdoor activities are very important to make an individual a complete person.It gives you the sense of accountability , Team spirit , Leadership quality and Motivation to achieve something in real life , to prove yourself as an individual in the society.Many times it has been observed that a good sports person is also good in academics and a good achiever in his work place.Better sports persons are quick and better decision maker in real life.There are plenty of examples. The one person coming in my mind immediately is none other than *"The owner of Dallas Mavericks "*,Mr. Mark Cuban.Its always recommended to be a part of some sports , that engages you with a huge group of people who also love the same sports and help you grow socially.

Healthy Sports :

Swimming : We already have discussed about it in the last chapter.As a sport swimming has several benefits.it keeps you at a healthy body weight,improves lung capacity and helps to build your muscles and burn callories.

Tennis: One hour of Tennis helps to burn 600 callories.The different body movements required in Tennis e.g pivot , slam , sprints etc help to achieve your body's core strength.

Aerobics: Aerobics are the strength training exercises that can also be considered as sports.It helps to achieve significant gain in overall fitness.Most of the important gain are Muscular strength , CardioVascular Improvement and flexibility.It is usually performed with music guided by an instructor.

Skiing : This is a really effective sport and burns more calorie than any other sports ,around 1100. skiing keeps you 40% fitter than other sports.

Volleyball : makes our list for healthiest sports because it increases metabolic rate, builds agility, strengthens coordination, and boosts mood, Oh, and it also burns plenty of calories.a person can burn between 90 to 133 calories during a half-hour

30

game of non-competitive, non-beach volleyball, depending on a person's weight, while a competitive gym game of volleyball burns between 120 to 178 calories.

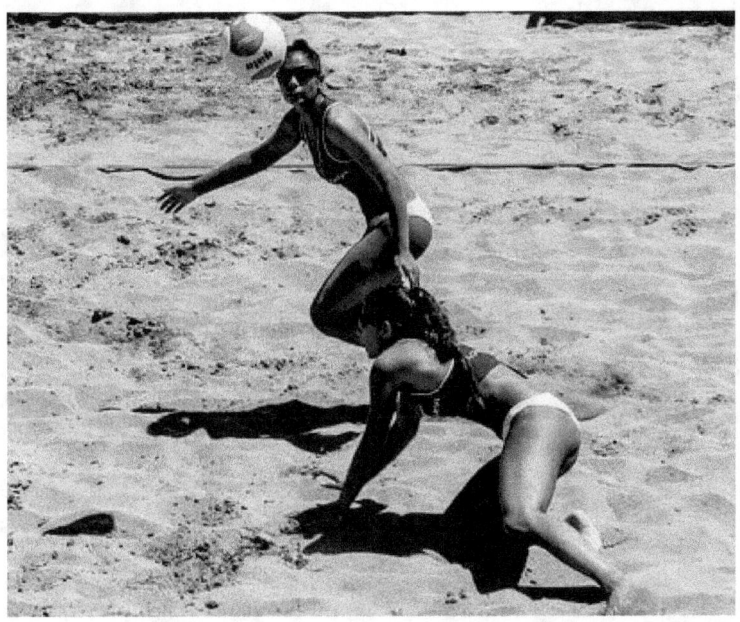

Gymnastics : Gymnastics is an amazing sports that keeps mind and body extremely flexible.Though its not easy to attain the skill and needs proper guidance from instructor but keeps our body in a really great shape.it is beneficial for improving concentration and mental focus. Gymnastics allows children the chance to think for themselves, to stimulate their imaginations and to solve problems safely.

Outdoor Activities :

Camping : Camping is one of the most fun thing to do when you have break from work. The best part is to suddenly get ready for it with friends and family and spend the time in an isolated place close to nature.It makes you unplugged, get rid of the everyday anxiety and stress and gives the kind of relief and satisfaction thats actually improve your mind and body fitness. Its adventurous and gives you the freedom to explore nature.Camping improves your sleep.

Hiking : Hiking is a really exercise for your body. Hiking gives the following benefits.Cardio Respiratory Fitness
- Muscle Fitness
- Lower the risk of heart disease and stroke
- Lower the risk of cancer specially breast , lung and colon cancer
- Weight Control
- Lower the risk of Early Death
- Burns about 350 calories

Hiking is really good for kids as well.If we can spend 2.5 hours a week thats enough to reduce the risk of cancer. In week days we can go to nearest spot near office for 10 mins hiking.

-

Fishing :

Full body workout : Fishing is a natural workout ,there by gaining lots of strength. Its fun and trying to catch even small fish also helps to improve entire body strength such as shoulder , legs , hips ,back muscle etc. It strengthen the muscle of arms.

Cardiovascular System :   Fishing is one kind of a fun adventure where you have to walk around to find the right spot and concentrate on catching the fish.Going for fishing and walking improve your cardiovascular system.It puts pressure on your heart and lungs.

Promotes Relaxation : Fishing is probably a whole day exercise. Sitting at a place close to nature ,far from the crowd and focusing on catching the fish relaxes your mind and body.It reduces anxiety and blood pressure.

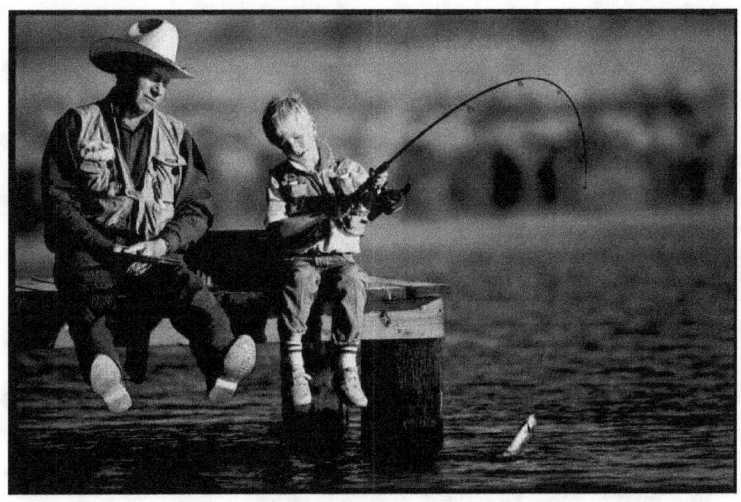

Family Fishing

Being Patience : Fishing helps to improve your skills to be patience.It makes you being patient a practice.

9

Chapter 7 : Social Engagement

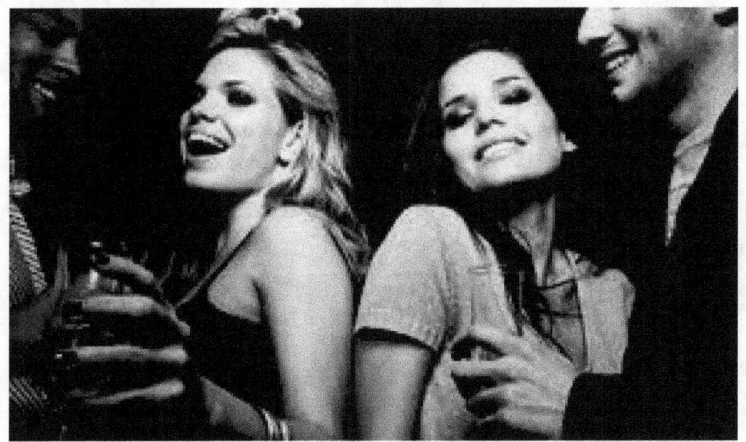

Human being is a social animal. Engaging into social activity is a part of life and it also promotes better Mental and Physical Health.Someone who is unsocial , introvert and doesn't want to participate into social activity slowly develops self centeredness , becomes selfish, develops the fear to express himself/herself , suffers from anxiety and depression.

Social Engagement can be done in different ways. Different countries have different cultures and different rituals. As a part of the active society we can take part into different cultural festival. We can participate into some activity or perform something on stage being a participant.This also develops our confidence as a person and make ourself a responsible social entity.When you realize that people have started noticing you then automatically we are concerned to live in a way that's healthier.We are concerned about our physical presence.

We can also engage ourself through different Social Meetups e.g Arts or painting Exhibition , Science Exhibition,singing competition etc.

Social Media

Social Media has become a predominant factor to keep us engaged into several social engagement. After the inception of powerful social platform like Facebook , Twitter almost every educated person in this world is able create his/her own social world.

In facebook we can be a part of an existing group or create our own group and invite people to nurture common interest. It provides the platform to connect people of similar interest e.g photography , Painting etc.

Social Events :

Its often recommended by doctors that drinking moderate alcohol socially improves heart condition than drinking none. In Todays busy world Clubbing ,Dancing etc are a another way to become social. It releases stress and dancing as a form of exercise improves our fitness.

Being in Relation:

It's easy to assume that a low-maintenance, drama-free romantic relationship should be relatively free of stress. To boot, there are studies to back that up.Recent studies have found that single people are more prone to psychological stress than those who are married or in a steady relationship. Relationship status can affect the production of cortisol, a stress hormone, during stressful events.Unmarried adults had a higher probability of early death than those who were married and living with their spouses.

   New relationships offer some particularly enthralling health boosts. In men, a new romantic partner can trigger the release of testosterone and dopamine, chemicals that can contribute to feelings of lust, attachment, and happiness — they also help your body recover and feel good.It gives you mental support ,more leisure hour ,more wealth.

10

Conclusion

Thanks For Reading my book. Hope I was able to convey sensible messages to all of you and you will really try to implement these habits to your life. Health is the first priority to become wealthy. We are so much into our everyday routine work that we sometimes forget whats good for us and whats not. Good sleep , Drinking lots of water ,Exercise,Sports & outdoor ,yoga and meditation and social involvement are unavoidable. If we don't provide these to our mind and body they won't help us to achieve what we really want in life and suddenly draw a full stop.Everyone is not fortunate enough in this world to have the luxury to achieve all the ways out to develop these habits but we have to figure out a way by ourselves. Just blaming the system or the society is not enough.We have to first take care of ourselves then only we can take care of others.I am stating this facts from my own experience and failures and want all of you to participate ,collaborate and make world a better place to live. Please share more information and your views. Shoot me an email any time and we can take it to the next level and create an awarness.Here is my email address

Email : jyotirmoydb@gmail.com
Website : www.theprecisecontent.com

11

References

- *http://www.mensjournal.com/expert-advice/10-health-benefits-of-being-in-a-relationship-20140904/get-taken-care-of*
- *http://www.yogajournal.com/article/health/count-yoga-38-ways-yoga-keeps-fit/*
- *https://www.artofliving.org/in-en/meditation/meditation-for-you/benefits-of-meditation*
- *http://www.healthfitnessrevolution.com/top-10-healthiest-sports/*
- *25 Reasons Running is Better than the Gym*